I0837375

The Chain Trick Part 1: Heroin

When I first posted this in May 2016, I had limited experience with the chain trick. I'm a little in awe at the creativity that SOMEONE had in coming up with this. I mean, think about it. How did that go the first time someone thought this up?

"C'mere sub! Lay down! I'm going to work several feet of heavy duty chain inside your cooter and then I'm gonna pull it out rather fast!"

"Yes, sir." (she says nervously envisioning the potential catastrophic damage to said cooter)

To me, it sounds like something a Master would do as a horrific sadistic punishment, and the discovery of its awesomeness was a happy accident. Serendipity! Which is something I'm 100% a fan of.

The first time I tried it, it was with SOB, (see previous stories). Her pussy was absolutely cavernous and we probably could have filled her with a considerable length of chain. And being a MASSIVE squirter, that show would have been one for the record books. Sadly, she chickened out with only about a few links inside her.

I also suggested it with Sunshine (also see previous stories). However, the look of sheer terror on her face told me that maybe she wasn't a good candidate for such experimental play. You know you've crossed a line when the look on a woman's face says, "My God. I am playing with a madman!" And she probably laid awake at night in fear of what demonic activities I was planning.

The ex wife was such an anal slut that it was a natural thing for us to try. We tried quite a few times. But, it always ended one of two ways. The first, I'd get a little chain into her, she'd cum and shoot the chain back out. A couple times, she damn near put my eye out with the end of that chain flying out of her ass towards my face. The other result was that it only turned her on ferociously and she'd beg me to fist her. And well, I kinda loved fisting her ass. I always figured we'd get it eventually. Sigh. I really miss playing with her ass. Not her. I don't miss HER at all. But I definitely miss shoving things up her ass.

Bama and I tried the chain. Pictures available by request. But as I said, I wasn't the most experienced at this and we had some pinching. Her vag is a wee bit shallow, too. It opens beautifully for my fist, but it doesn't have a lot of depth. So, the amount of chain I got into her was deceptive. Really, only about 12", I'm guessing. She said she liked it, although it didn't really rock her world. "Maybe if there was more of it in there to pull out," she said. We have vowed to try again.

I had an opportunity to try with another woman later, but it didn't work out. I discovered that she had screaming, intense orgasms when I fingered and rimmed her ass. I LOVE THAT!! Hey, have you heard the one about the two old guys walking in the woods? They come upon a frog on the side of the path. The frog says, "Kiss me and I'll turn into a beautiful princess." One of the guys picks the frog up and slips it into his pocket. The other guy says, "Morty! What are you doing? It's a beautiful princess!" Morty shrugs and says, "At my age, Bernie, I'd rather have a talking frog." THIS was kinda like that!! So, we forgot all about the chain trick and I spent most of the weekend fingering and rimming her ass.

A couple of times, I tried it with a man. I had a fisting student a while back that agreed to try it. We had not quite managed to get my big ol' fist into his ass yet. But, we had done some nice work with a few toys - one was a 18" double dildo that I managed to slowly work all the way into him. The session previous, I sent him home that way and instructed him to leave it until his wife got home from work later and let her remove it while sucking him off. That was quite a few years ago and he still thanks me for that.

Anyway. I digress. We tried the chain on him. But sadly, we encountered one of the challenges of the trick. The pinching. It's hard! You have to be very careful and proceed very slowly. The tighter the orifice, the more challenging. Pushing link after link, into a tight asshole, some pinching was to be expected. He decided after a few times, that maybe the chain trick wasn't for him. I had to let him have that one.

Another man, an experienced fistee, could open up impressively and take a fist like few I've ever met. When I suggested the chain trick, his eyes lit up. "I've always wanted to try that!!" So, we did. The first time, we used a smaller chain than the one pictured. And, because he could open up so well for fisting, we tried an unconventional technique to avoid the pinching. I would fill my hand with chain, shove my fist inside him, open my hand and deposit the chain, pull my hand out for more chain. Repeat until the entire 3-1/2' we had were inside him with just enough to grip for the finale. Saying that he liked it would be an understatement. It took him a little while to collect himself, ass up, face down, damn near hyperventilating with a death grip on the sheets.

After a little aftercare, gently caressing his ass cheeks and legs, he whispered, "Can we do it again?"

"Found your heroin, have we?"

He could only nod. We did it three times that afternoon and each time I knew he had gone to a special place. You know how it is. Once you cross a line and enter a place like that, there is no coming back. Nothing else will satisfy the same way again. It's the fuel of obsession. This man was there. I knew his life was changed forever. Even fisting - which had previously been his heroin - now had a spot in the back seat (no pun intended).

The next time we tried it, he showed up with some more substantial chain. See pictures. "Can we do it with this this time?"

I smiled. "If you want" I answered as nonchalant as I could. Secretly though, I was thinking about a thicker chain anyway, and this was the same chain I had used on Bama and the other woman. Great minds thinking alike, I guess. The ex wife and I also tried the thicker chain and I told you how that went. LOL. So, I was excited to try it with this guy.

I warmed him up with my fingers and then some toys, gradually working up to some larger toys. I fisted him thoroughly for about 15 minutes, going as deep as he could handle (which is about midway up my forearm). When I felt he was sufficiently prepped, I began lubing up the chain. This guy is particular to good ol' Crisco. I slathered a thick coating on the chain and began to insert it. Because the chain was twice as thick, I could only put half as many in my fist at a time. It took a while. And, it made my fist considerably larger to slip in. He grunted a little each time I shoved into him.

Slowly, patiently, I kept putting more chain into him. Before I realized it, I had worked about 5-1/2' feet inside!! I don't know where it went, but he was running out of room. I tried to ever so gently push it along a little but got some pinching and resistance. I figured we had reached his limit for the day.

I was also starting to grow concerned about the weight inside him. I could only estimate, but I was thinking we were somewhere in the thirty pounds range. That CANNOT be healthy for any part of a person's colon, anal cavity, etc. I had visions of driving him to an emergency room and having to explain to a room full of horrified nurses what we'd been up to. I know. I know. Emergency room nurses have seen it all. Buuuuuutttt... I'm betting several feet of heavy duty chain would be a first for many of them.

I asked if he was ready. His breathing got quick as he nodded. I smiled. I had a feeling this was going to be a new high for him. Very quickly, I pulled 2 links out. He gasped. I almost laughed. This was going to be epic!!

"Squeeze," I told him. "Not too tight, but try to hold it in."

"Oh my God," he moaned just above a whisper as I tugged slightly to test for the tightness.

"Here we go," I said calmly. He grasped the sheets and dug in. He took a deep breath as I began to pull. Briskly, but not too fast. I was still feeling some caution as I pulled. His body quivered violently as the chain came out. He buried a scream into the bed that lasted until a full 15 seconds after the chain was completely out of him. I dared not touch him, allowing his orgasm to subside naturally. Two. Three minutes went by. His fists still clenched the sheets, and I wasn't sure he had taken a breath. I lightly ran my hand across his ass cheek. He gasped and shook again. Just out of meanness, I guess, I shoved my fist back into him and gave it a few quick, hard thrusts. I thought he was going to lose it. He screamed again, this time not into the bed.

"No more," he he begged. "No more. Please." Every time I even breathed in his direction, he quivered uncontrollably and begged me to stop. I did as he asked and even moved away to let him return to earth. I'm not sure if he dozed off, but he became very still and calm. I watched carefully to make sure he was still breathing. Mostly though, I just patiently waited.

Years ago, I was going down on a woman, Susan, and I made her hyperventilate so bad we had to call 9-1-1. See, I have this gap between my front two teeth that allows me to just kinda "lock on" to a woman's clit. Depending on the size and shape of her clit, of course. I use my arms to hold her legs up and she's really stuck. She breathlessly told me to stop. I didn't. In fact, I intensified my tongue action. I thought I was being funny. I thought, after she catches her breath, she'll thank me for pushing her to a new level of ecstasy. I was wrong.

She literally couldn't breath. Not quite turning blue, but still scary. Making the call, I just told the operator that she couldn't catch her breath without elaborating on what led to our current situation. I tried to dress her while we waited, but she wasn't having any part of me touching her or helping her.

Of course, the paramedics were two women. They demanded that I explain what led to a naked woman in my bed not being able to breath. I don't know. Maybe thinking I had drugged her or done something unsavory, or possibly illegal to her. So, I thought, "What the hell?" and I told them. One of the women rolled her eyes and turned away. The other one locked eyes with me like she was trying to determine if I was fucking with them or not. I shrugged and nodded. "It's true."

She shook her head in disbelief and they checked out my lady friend. She was fine. In fact, by the time they arrived, she'd already started getting her wits back. As they were leaving, the second paramedic slipped me her number and whispered, out of earshot of her partner, "If I die, my husband can't find out."

Susan never let me eat her again, not willingly anyway. Next time I went down on her, she broke up with me afterwards. "You almost killed me asshole! I ain't got time for that!" Oh well.

So anyway. I left the guy alone and let him collect his senses. After what seemed like forever, he said, "Fuck."

"Back from heaven?"

He shook his head and said, "Fuck" again.

"Ready to go again?" I asked, joking of course.

"NO!!" he hollered. "You touch me again, it'll probably kill me." He rolled over onto his side, eyes still closed, just a puddle of flesh at that point. I still didn't touch him; just watched. And waited. And waited. And waited. I got some water and handed him the bottle. Condensation dripped on to his hand and he shook hard. He drank half the bottle at once and handed it back to me, unsure about holding it himself. Slowly, he tried to prop himself up on the pillows. It was a challenge. Seriously. But he finally made it. Only then did he open his eyes. When he did, I could tell. Something was different.

Fuck," he said again. He shook his head and stared at me.

"I'm guessing it was good?" I asked. "I've never seen ANYONE zone out like that after an orgasm."

He reached for the water again and I handed it to him. He drank most of the remainder before he answered. I quote, "I saw God." He shook his head and started to try and explain, but every time he opened his mouth, nothing came out. He killed the last of the water and said, "That wasn't just an orgasm. I think I literally left my body."

Well, I didn't have an answer for that at the time, so I just watched him. He was still shaky and didn't seem like he was entirely "back" yet. I usually kick guys out when I'm done with them. But, I had to let this one sleep a while.

When he emerged from the bedroom three hours later, still on unsteady legs, I offered him food and he ate a little soup. Not much. Said, he couldn't handle much. Every time I touched him, he flinched a little and quivered. It was really hard not to dance and pound my chest, boasting. I've given women plenty of orgasms. PLENTY!! But to this day, no woman had ever said she left her body, though. It really was a proud moment for me.

I didn't talk to him again for a while. Maybe 3 months. Maybe four. I texted him and asked if he'd been avoiding me. I told him "My fist misses you. LOL"

He texted back, "I'm retired." Followed by, "At least for a while."

I asked what he meant. He answered that he'd been to the mountain top. "That was so intense that it scared the fuck outta me." Followed by, "I don't wanna know where that train goes."

"LIke heroin?"

"YYYYYYYYYY" he answered.

After that, I have not talked to him. I tried to text him before I started writing this and he never answered. I'm never sure what that means.

The Chain Trick Part 2: Basic Information

Since posting my story about my experience with the chain trick, I have had several conversations about chaining. And, my experience with it has grown significantly. For this update, I'd like to share some of the content of those conversations and experiences in the addendum to this post.

Originally, I bought coated chain at Lowe's, for about $4-5 per foot. Figuring that this would be a session that would be unforgettable, $20-$25 seemed like a small price to pay.

The non coated chain had burrs at the seams and I imagined that being incredibly painful for the chainee. Shopping at local hardware stores, I could not find uncoated chain that didn't have the burrs and seam issues.

The first time, I used a chain that was half as thick/heavy. But after, I went up to the larger chain size, thinking fewer links, and larger links, would reduce the likelihood of pinching. Not sure if I was right or not. They both seemed to have SOME pinching because there is a significant learning curve to putting the chain inside.

The coating seems to be a vinyl of some kind. I couldn't find more of a description. I imagine the manufacturer probably doesn't recommend "internal use". But, the coating seemed to survive SINGLE uses without chipping or peeling or wear. I did not dare use the same chain twice, thinking after the first time, the coating was a virtual petri dish of bacteria that I couldn't guarantee to sanitize it to anyone's comfort.

For fisting, the chain trick and any kind of large insertions where a heavy dose of lube is prescribed, I personally like grapeseed oil, coconut oil and EVOO for lube. It is generally safe for the body, with very few people having any kind of reaction to it. Some, of course, but very few. It has a tremendous amount of "slipperyness" and doesn't absorb into the tissue right away like many water-based lubes. It makes a mess and you have to consider, before you play, that it will possibly go everywhere. But other than that, it has worked well for me.

A LOT of people depend on plain ol' Crisco for this type of play. It also works great. And the handful (no pun intended) of men who have had my fist in them, most of them brought their own can.

There are also many designer lubes on the market. Some people swear by them. For me though, they either dry out and have to be reapplied too often or they don't provide the same amount of lubrication as the oils. That is just MY experience with it. If you have something that works for you, carry on.

That said, many lubes can wear the coatings off some cheap toys. If you have a dildo or vibrator that has turned colors or has discolored spots, throw it out!! The coating on the chain seemed to survive the first use. However, I would be nervous about a second use. I wasn't sure how much the oil penetrated the coating. Like I said, ANY use like this could turn the chain into a petri dish of bacteria. I never considered using the chain a second time or with a second person.

I also know that anything used to clean the chain could compromise the coating. Even mild soap and warm water could possibly break it down. I wasn't sure, and I didn't want to risk it. Safety first, right? Plus, cleaning the chain, link by link, seemed like a horribly tedious task. I'd rather buy a new chain. It's inexpensive.

In these conversations, someone let me know about McMaster-Carr. They have smooth, stainless steel chain available on their website. It is definitely more expensive than the variety from Lowe's ($6-$9 ft). BUT, because this would be reusable, it actually saves money. And, no need to worry about the coating.

I spoke to someone at McMaster-Carr about their chain. The agent confirmed that the chain is flush on the outside, but on the inside, there is a slight "undulation" that keeps the chain from moving around very much (which might help with the pinching). He didn't actually look at a piece of the chain, but has talked to others about this and says the undulation is smooth and should not have any sharp edges. Not wanting to try and explain the chain trick over the phone, I told him it was for an art project and that people would be handling the chain, and we didn't want our hands cut up. He said this should work perfectly. :)

The link (no pun intended) to McMaster-Carr where some good chain is available:

http://www.mcmaster.com/#Standard-Stainless-Steel-Chain

I have not tried their twisted link chain. However, I can see the possibility that it would possibly reduce some of the pinching. Maybe. No reason to think that, other than my own gut reaction when I saw it.

The Chain Trick Part 3: Experience Update

Since posting this series in 2016, I had the opportunity to add to my experience over the next year. I ordered 6' each of 3/8" chain and 5/8" chain from McMaster-Carr. Less than $100 total, including shipping.

The nice thing was that I could reuse the chain. Right before a session, I soaked it in the sink, in regular dish soap, for about an hour or two. I used my hand to quickly wash each link. Then, I put it in the dishwasher. No soap. After the dishwasher finished, I'd open the door for about 1/2 hour and the chain was ready to use. Being still warm, but not hot.

In addition to the few mentioned in the previous story, I met with 11 women for vaginal chaining. Of those, 2 tried it anally after having some great results vaginally. Experience is definitely a plus. Each time, the session went a little better. I got better at reducing the pinching and seemed to find the sweet spot for how fast to pull the chain out. There seems to be a "Goldilocks Zone" for that, balancing too much intensity and not enough. None of them claimed to "see God" like the man in the previous story. But when I found the right speed to yank the chain out, those women squirted mightily and had an orgasm they'll never forget.

For 8 of those women, we used the 3/8" chain. For the other 3, we used the 5/8" chain.

The two that tried it anally, they were experienced with anal sex and anal fisting, with an enthusiastic level of enjoyment with larger anal insertions. Both were well familiar with anal orgasms. For both, we engaged in a brief anal fisting session until they had an orgasm, and then took a short break before we attempted the chaining. We tried it twice, with each size chain, with each woman able to hold about 24"-30" of chain before they felt "full".

Both of the women experienced a wonderful orgasm with the 3/8" chain, and that it is definitely something they will do again. But when we tried the larger chain, it felt nice, but no orgasm. Possibly, because by that time, after some toy play and the short fisting session and the first chaining session, there was some fatigue and tenderness. Probably.

And then, right before everything went to shit in Knoxville, I was also visited by a lovely woman from Vancouver named Marina. She brought her submissive girlfriend, Tanya. They were in Knoxville for an art installation (Knoxville is actually a very artsy town, believe it or not) and we got a glorious opportunity to experiment with the chain trick quite a few times while they were in town. Neither was brave enough to try it anally, even though they had fisted each other anally regularly. Vaginal chaining and fisting was wide open though.

Marina, a tall, slender woman was able to hold almost 5' of the smaller chain and about 3' of the larger chain. Tanya, a smaller woman, was able to comfortably hold slightly less, but not a lot less. We made it a true science project and tried all kinds of variations to find different ways of inserting the chain and the climactic moment of pulling it out.

All together over a two-week span, Mariana got chained about 25 times and Tanya about 30. Each woman had orgasms most times that we pulled it out. Most of the time, they squirted quite a bit, even when they didn't have an orgasm.

Which brings us to the first thing we learned. It takes time to insert the chain. Even when a woman pees and fully empties her bladder BEFORE we begin, by the time we are ready to pull the chain out, they might need to pee again. Since the chain puts pressure on the urethral sponge inside her, and those links hit the sponge coming out, it should be expected that there might be some urination simultaneous to the ejaculation.

Now, if you've read my volumes of squirting, you know that ejaculation IS NOT urine and they DO NOT exit the body from the same place. Urine exits through the urethra. Ejaculation exits through the paraurethra, or ducts of the Skene's Glands. Urine and ejaculate are not the same thing. HOWEVER, the urethral sponge controls their exit from the body for both. So, extreme stimulation of the kind with chaining, can cause both when the urethral sponge is so heavily stimulated.

Just a warning. Be prepared. We used an outdoor tarp under the women while we were doing all this, in part to catch the bodily fluids, but also to accommodate so much lube going everywhere.

Second thing we learned is that there is also a sweet spot for the angle of pulling the chain out. Pulling the chain out straight away in line with the vaginal canal was nice and brought them to orgasm most times. It had the extreme stimulation to the urethral sponge and g-spot, causing great squirting and pleasure.

BUT, when we pulled up SLIGHTLY as the chain was pulled out, we got the added benefit of the chain stimulating the clit. I want to emphasize that I raised the angle JUST SLIGHTLY.

Too much was too rough on the poor clit and caused soreness as well as pressure on the pubic bone and upper entrance to the vagina. With each woman, there was a slight variation in the perfect angle. With your partner, you'll need to experiment to find the sweet spot for you/her.

And, we experimented with body positions. On her back, knees raised, feet down, was definitely the best position.

- This seemed to allow the most chain to be inserted for some reason. On all fours, the weight of the chain made each woman say she was full a little sooner.

- On her back, there seemed to be more forgiveness for a bad angle or a less than perfect extraction.

- Because of the time it takes to insert a considerable length of chain into her body, there was also a fatigue factor of knees, back, arms, neck, etc. Who knew doggy style, just staying in that position for a while, while someone inserted some chain into your girl parts would be physically uncomfortable after a while?

- And last, when she's on her back, the person putting the chain in can stimulate her clit with mouth, fingers or toys. This is not really an option when she's on her knees.

Our grand finale was a couple of experiments on Marina. The first one, Tanya and I BOTH inserted a chain into her (the smaller and larger chains) and pulled them out at the same time. If there was ever a moment that she might have had a spiritual experience, I think that was it. The squirting and orgasm was epic. She needed aftercare. Tanya held her about 45 minutes until she got her wits back and was ready to try the second experiment.

The second experiment was for Tanya and I to insert both ends of both chains, thus pulling out FOUR chains simultaneously. We had low expectations, anticipating soreness and fatigue by that point. But, it went well. Not even close to as big as the previous experiment, but it took the rest of the day to get the smile off Marina's face. I'm thinking that meant she liked it.

As for men, I got MANY messages from men who said they also wanted to try it and see God, but only a few actually showed up for our appointments. I've noticed that this seems to be a common result with arranging playdates of ANY kind with men. They're home alone, watching porn, get turned on and think they want something, but before they actually arrive, they chicken out.

In conversations with men who have tried chaining, the reviews were varied. Some REALLY liked it. Some really DID NOT. Most were somewhere in the middle. It was okay, somewhat pleasurable, but no one left their bodies or anything like that.

Well, four men showed up. Two, we tried it and they liked it. One had an orgasm, one didn't. Both were more impressed with fisting though. Both said they got impatient with the time it took to insert the chain. Kinda lost their horniness. For each of them, we tried it twice, smaller chain and larger chain. Always the same report.

The other two brought their Domme with them. The first, he wanted to warm up with some pegging and fisting. So, she worked him over for a while. But after that, he had already had a couple of orgasms and had lost interest in the chain at that point.

A fifth man though, he was fun. He told me in his messages that he is multi-orgasmic and his colon can go all night without getting sore or tired. I laughed and thought, 'Challenge accepted'.

We began with some toys and got his initial orgasm out of the way. That seemed to just get him more turned on though, which is what I hoped. I fisted him for over an hour, sometimes slow and deep and sometimes, hard and fast. And as he promised, he was truly multi-orgasmic. I was impressed. There are quite a few men online who claim to be multi-orgasmic through Tantra practices, who teach about male internal orgasms. I've talked to quite a few men who claim they have experienced that. This was the first time I'd seem it in person though.

When we got to the chain, I asked if he wanted to take a break first. With a big smile, he said, "Go for it!" So, we started with the smaller chain. After about 4', I pulled it out and he moaned pleasantly. He said he came, but fisting was better. So, we tried the bigger chain, with me inserting it with my fist. That was much better he said, but the part he liked best was my hand going in an out. So, I fisted him until my arms were exhausted and he left quite happy.

Everyone wanted the extreme spiritual experience I described in the first story. And while most people thought chaining was awesome and an experience they'll never forget, none experienced anything spiritual. I was disappointed. And even the ones who thoroughly enjoyed it, it was probably a little disappointing for them too. Whether the experience lived up to the hype is a matter of opinion.

If you think about how an orgasm works, a spiritual experience makes perfect sense. Orgasm is actually NOT a physiological event; it is a cerebral one. The euphoria you feel when you cum is the release of chemicals in the brain. Oxytocin (my favorite), Serotonin, Dopamine, and a few others. It is a bit of a learned response to the physical stimulation. The brain says, "Do that to the body as the cause and the effect is orgasm", and it triggers the release of the chemicals as the appropriate response. We all have a pretty standard process and a fairly standard amount of chemicals released.

But, if you're REALLY, REALLY turned on and do something special to the body, it is possible that the brain will OVER-release those chemicals, making that orgasm a special one. Just my theory on that. There is no research on it that I've found.

In a very special case, when you think about chakras and the third eye and all the spirituality of sexual release, "seeing God" doesn't seem as crazy as it sounds. Since the event, I have experimented with a few women who were REALLY into yoga and chakras to see if we could make them "see God". We worked on a lot of teasing and edging to bring their arousal higher and higher so that when they finally had their orgasm, it was a very special one. Although an unforgettable orgasm, so far, no such luck with seeing God. Although, that could just be a matter of semantics because of the way they described an orgasm that over-the-top, far beyond a regular orgasm.

I also asked them if they felt like they left their body for a moment, after explaining the question. Most said they understood how he might have felt that way, but "No. I didn't leave my body." Sigh.

Personally, chaining is such an extreme, awesome, uncommon thing to do, I can't wait to find someone to do it regularly with. If you're out there, message me!!

The Happy Hand Part 1: The Greeter

I talk a big game about fisting. I have lots of experience and lots of love for it. Those of you who have been following me since the pre-FetLife days probably remember that my previous moniker was FunWithFists. Good times. Good times.

Personally, I believe it's as intimate as it gets between two people because of the level of trust and communication it takes for a successful session. It's not my primary kink. But, it's possibly one of the things I have the most experience with. So, I thought I would start with how and where I got into it.

My first paying photo gig was of body piercing. It wasn't a huge paycheck, and I didn't get the byline. But it was my first paycheck as a professional photographer. The photographer that was assigned the gig didn't want it. "I'm not spending a week with those weirdos!" he said. I emphatically volunteered. I needed that first check to get my career off the ground. AND, I WANTED to spend a week with those weirdos. I thought that would be as interesting as it gets.

So, I spent a week with the weirdos. A well-known piercer had offered to be the host and subject of the story. He introduced me and the writer of the story part to many people in the D.C. area who had some unique piercings and equally unique stories behind those piercings. It was the freakiest thing I'd ever seen up to that point in my life. I saw people with things pierced in ways that made me think, "WHAT THE FUCK!?!" I saw things I can never UNsee. This is before I'd ever heard of O'Pearl (maybe even before her extreme career got started, I don't know). Since, I've seen some unbelievable piercings and body modifications that were even more unbelievable. But at that time, this was the freakiest shit I could imagine.

One of the questions I kept asking was, "WHY?" I mean, in my opinion, the human body has a certain number of holes that all perform a specific function. The human body does not need any extra holes, especially holes that don't perform some kind of biological purpose. That was, until I hung out with these people for a week and realized that they aren't any more weird than anyone else.

They all told me that I'd never really understand until I got something pierced. But once I did, I'd understand completely without a word being said. By the end of the week, I got open-minded. I couldn't pierce an ear because I dealt with very conservative people and I didn't think it would fly. I was NOT about to pierce my privates. Belly button? Well, that's for teenage girls. So, I decided a nipple was the thing to do.

FUUUUUUUUUUCCCCK!!!! There are no words to describe the pain. Not just the pain of getting it done, but the pain of snagging it on a shirt a week later. The pain of the seatbelt in the car damn near slicing off my perpetually erect nipple. The pain of the first time I bumped it on something. The pain of turning over in my sleep. You just aren't aware of how much nipples move around until you get one pierced.

I thought about taking it out every single day. Two things prevented me. The first was that I was starting to get what no one could explain. The second was that I'd already crossed the Rubicon. My nipple was going to take time to heal, with or without the piercing. I may as well leave it in.

What I was starting "to get" was the mental and emotional rewards of the pierced nipple. The first was a cool factor. We all have things about us that are cool and beautiful. Most days, I feel pretty good about myself. But on those other days, I'll feel the nipple ring (I soon got a seamless ring that I still hang baubles from) and I will feel just a little cooler and sexier than that day's self esteem would allow. I can feel it under my shirt, rubbing, and I know I am just a little sexier and cooler than mere mortals who do not have a nipple pierced.

The second is the empowerment. If I can handle getting a nipple pierced, I can handle anything. On my scariest days, I remember that and it gets me through.

Well, the host for the photo gig, a man named Valentine (pronounced Val-en-TEEN), was obviously who I was going to have do the piercing. So, I called him up. Apparently, he did this from his home. That's not scary at all, ya know. But, I went over to his place and had it done.

His house is this huge old house in the historic district with three stories and a basement (which I later found out was the dungeon). Walking in, I saw everything imaginable for BDSM. I saw a dog crate in a corner of the foyer WITH A WOMAN IN IT CURLED UP SLEEPING, just like a dog would. I saw several people walking around naked, a couple that were on leashes pulled around by a Master of some kind. Valentine met me in the foyer and told me to ignore his guests. "Hard to do that," I mumbled.

He waved me to the back of the house where he performed the piercings. Already, I was questioning how smart I was for going there. I talked with this guy for an entire week and had no idea he had all that going on. Not one word. But now that the secret was out, he told me about his BDSM activities as he was setting up for the piercing. Turned out, he was quite the character in the local BDSM community. Presumably, still is.

"You should come to one of my parties," he offered. "It'll be a wild night you'll never forget."

By this time, the curiosity was getting to me. And, as a lifelong student of all things sexual, I figured I NEEDED to experience this. So, I agreed to attend. When the piercing was complete, I left.

When party night came around, I brought a friend who I knew was pretty adventurous. We parked and walked up to the door. From the outside, the house looked like any other house on the block. A VERY nice old house, but just like all the other nice old houses. I don't know what I expected, but with the hype, I didn't expect it to look "normal". I thought, maybe, some extra lights, or a marquee or something.

A naked young nymph of a woman opened the door. She had an uncountable number of facial piercings. She didn't appear to even be of legal age. My friend and I looked at each other like, "Holy shit! Are we sure we want to go in?" But before we could chicken out, Valentine dragged us inside and gave us each a full on bear hug.

"Welcome!!" he shouted.

I couldn't answer. Right there in the foyer, there was a big sturdy wooden table. On that table was a naked man, ass up, face down with his head in a big wooden box. His arms were bound to the table straight out to his sides and his ankles were bound in place to keep him from going anywhere. On the table next to his knees was a selection of oversized toys. There was a dildo that had to be 18" in length and the diameter of my arm. There were a variety of buttplugs of different sizes. There was a Nerf football. You heard me. A Nerf football. The item that unsettled me most was the electric wand. Also on the table was a ginormous pump bottle of lube and a box of elbow length gloves.

"Oh," Valentine waved his hand at the man on the table. "Say 'Hello' to Norman. He's our greeter."

While my friend and I stood there pondering how exactly we were supposed to say hello to a man bound in such a way, ass up, face down on a table in the foyer, a couple came in and demonstrated. The woman picked up the wand, switched it on and began swabbing the inside of the man's gaping anus with it. I could hear him screaming, even with his head inside the box. That was so disturbing, I almost screamed along with the poor guy. The woman giggled and stepped aside so her date could say hello. He chose the Nerf football and roughly shoved it all the way into the man's ass and just left it there. The couple giggled and walked on into the party. My friend and I just stood there in complete disbelief.

"Go ahead," Valentine encouraged. "Say 'Hello'."

"What do we do?" I asked. "Just shove something up his ass?"

There was a man standing next to the table. A Sergeant At Arms of some kind, I presume, or a supervisor of some kind making sure the man wasn't violated too badly, or in an unapproved way. "Yep, anything here." he said like P.T. Barnum waving at the chance for a blowjob from the bearded lady. As he spoke, he yanked the Nerf football out of the man's ass and dropped it back on the table. "Or, if you want, just shove your ol' fist into him."

I did a double-take. "Excuse me?"

"Like this," he said as he put a glove on and shoved not just his fist, but his whole arm, elbow deep into the man's ass. Just shoved it right in. The man on the table barely made a sound. It was almost like he ENJOYED it.

"D-D-D-Does he even know we're back here?"

"Not a clue," Valentine laughed. "He has headphones on inside there."

I can only imagine the poor man on the table. There he is, all vulnerable and whatnot, and ALL OF A SUDDEN, there's something enormous being inserted into a place where enormous things should NEVER be inserted.

"HELLLLLLLOOOO!!!!!"

"And... He WANTED this?" I asked in disbelief. My friend was already shaking his head.

Valentine was nodding. "Yep. He volunteers for the job for every party."

By this time, another couple had entered. Two middle-aged women. After a quick hug and greeting from Valentine, they both grabbed some gloves and simultaneously shoved their fists into his ass. When they reached as deep as they could together, they pulled them out and took turns fisting the poor man for a few strokes. I swear I could hear the man moaning, and looking closely, I saw that he was leaking a little precum. Now, I wasn't just shocked, I was intrigued.

I went over and grabbed a glove. After a moment of consideration, I slipped the glove on and gently slid my hand inside. I could feel everything. I slowly slid it in almost to my elbow before it felt like I hit bottom. I heard the man moan as I pulled my hand back.

"Give him a few deep strokes. Don't deprive him," Valentine told me. I did. Each time, I was a little more fascinated with how this was biologically possible. My friend opted for the enormous dildo and gave the man a few deep strokes before giggling as he put the toy back on the table.

We walked through the party and saw more things I cannot UNsee. Not saying I want to UNsee those things. I'm just saying that the sights were a little overwhelming. Valentine walked through with us and explained each scene to us as we came to it, like a guide at a museum of art. I guess it was art in a way.

We saw a woman with her arms bound behind her and her ankles bound together tightly, hung from the ceiling by her hair. Clothes pins all over her. She was just hanging there like an exhibit. We saw another woman on a table tied in a pretzel with what I guessed was about a mile of rope. Her pussy was getting punch fisted by a very large angry woman. We saw another woman tied to a bench getting gangbanged. We saw a MAN tied to a bench across the room also getting gangbanged. And in the middle of all this, dozens of people were socializing, enjoying drinks and hors-d'oeuvres like nothing at all was going on around them.

We came to the glory hole. Basically, a make-shift sheetrock wall about 6 feet wide, and a little over six feet tall, anchored in place by heavy bolts and metal braces. "Go ahead," Valentine encouraged. I peeked behind the wall for a second and saw an attractive woman on her knees, blindfolded, with her Master's hand shoving her head to the hole to receive whatever came through. We watched about 10 minutes as 4 different guys came over and fucked her mouth vigorously before shooting a load down her throat.

"Thank you," she said to each one after they finished and pulled their cocks out. Cum ran down her chin, all over her breasts, down her body and puddled on the floor. I don't know how many loads she'd taken at that point, but it was clear that those weren't the first 4 guys.

I admit, part of me wanted to be next. But, I felt sorry for her. I felt sadness at what had to be some kind of terrible punishment. I know NOW that she probably wanted to be right there to serve her master or she was getting a tremendous amount of pleasure from it and would stay all night if he wanted her to, and would be entirely HAPPY to do so. I didn't know that THEN, or I might have taken a turn.

Valentine continued the tour downstairs. There was a medical room. There were people in stocks and strapped to a variety of things getting whipped and flogged. There were several rooms with naked people in dog cages and nothing else.

Another room had a very large guy bent over very far with his hands tied behind his back, tied to a rope from the celling forcing him to stay in that position. His legs and butt were covered in whelps from a beating. He had a hood on, but I could still hear him breathing hard. There were a couple of rooms for bodily fluids. He allowed us to peek through a window in the door. We didn't stay there but a second and I can safely say I wish I could UNsee what was going on in there.

My friend went mingling. He told me later he went back and took a turn at the glory hole. I was fascinated by the greeter though. I went back and just watched. I talked to the Sergeant at Arms about it. Apparently, the man on the table was his sub and he was there to protect him.

"Protect him?" I asked. "Well, I would think that would start by getting him off the table."

"Oh, no. You don't understand. This is what he wants."

I couldn't imagine ANYONE wanting a fist shoved up their ass. After it seemed like all that were going to show up had shown up, the Master released his sub. As he unbolted the box, allowing him to come up for air, I saw that the man was smiling from ear to ear. "How many?" he asked.

"Sixty one," the Master answered. And the man's grin got even bigger. "I think this guy wants to talk to you. You have permission."

"Hi," the man said cheerfully.

"Hi," I answered, not sure where to begin. "Sooooo... You WANTED to do this?"

"Oh, I love it," he answered. And then he turned to his Master, "Thank you, by the way." The Master nodded his approval.

"You're kidding, right?"

"No, I LOOOOOOOOOVE getting fisted. The other things are fine, but the feeling of the fist is what I truly love." He went on to explain how intimate it is because he can feel everything so intensely that way. I asked if he had "issues" afterwards. He explained that he'd been training his body for years to do this exact thing like an Olympic athlete. "For a few hours, I'm pretty loose back there. But by morning, I'm back to normal."

To say I was shocked after what I saw is an understatement. I flat out thought the guy was lying. There is NO WAY things went back to normal after that kind of attention. He assured me he was fine.

Valentine came over then. I asked him to confirm what the man told me and he did. "Yep. Tomorrow morning, he'll be fine."

"How is that possible?" I wondered. "I mean, what I saw just isn't biologically possible."

Valentine laughed. "Not for you," he said. "It's not a first date sort of thing, either. He's been working up to this for years."

I just looked at him. Stunned. "Teach me," I said before I realized what was coming out of my mouth.

"Really?" he asked, surprised. "You don't seem like a 'I'd like a fist up my ass kind of guy'. But then again, I wouldn't have expected you to get your nipple pierced, either."

"NOOOOO!!" I exclaimed. "Teach me how to do that to someone."

"Oh, that's easy to arrange." And that's how Valentine's Fisting School started. Okay, it wasn't an actual school. But every time I had some time, he would arrange some of his subs who were into being fisted to be available. And some of other Masters' subs. He taught me about anatomy and what to do once I got my fist inside. There's a bit of etiquette to it. There's some art to it. Some of the experienced subs were a wealth of knowledge. They taught me what felt good. And, what didn't. I got to practice a couple times a week for months. Men. Women. Vaginal. Anal. By myself and with someone else. It was an amazing education.

And that's how I got started. I haven't talked to Valentine since about '97. But, I still remember what he taught me. And since, I have learned a few tricks of my own by getting creative. I'm always creative. Gotta keep it interesting, ya know.

Story 1

When I was learning about fisting at Valentine's Fisting School, there was a lesbian woman who was only 19. She had never had a cock inside her, not even once. The most she'd ever had was a couple of WOMEN'S fingers.

Her Domme dropped her in my lap for me to practice on. When I first started, her pussy was so tight that it cut the circulation off when I only had three fingers inside her. Valentine promised me it would work if I took my time. Her Domme told her to stay with me until the job was done.

So, we worked on it for an hour. Took a break. Had some lunch and tried again for about an hour. I got four fingers in and she was fine. But from two hours of trying, her little pussy was getting VERY tender.

So, we stopped and went to a movie. We had coffee after. We sat at the coffee shop for a couple hours and laughed about life. Then, we came back and tried again. Ten minutes later, I was in. Changed her life.

Valentine, and the Domme, told me to always remember that it isn't that the fist won't fit in a vagina. A vagina is designed to stretch to allow an 8 pound bowling ball to exit. It might take work and it will allays take patience. But, it will always fit. They told me that the problem is believing that it will fit. Sometimes, you have to turn the hand a different way. Sometimes, you need more lube. But it will always fit.

Story 2

At a party a few months later, Valentine set up a fisting demonstration and I got to be the Master for it. On the big table that The Greeter was on at a previous party, there was a man. Next to him was his wife. Both of them were ass up and face down, asses facing me.

The man had an enormous piercing through his nut sack and it bolted to one side of the table. His dick had a Prince Albert piercing. It was stretched to its limit and bolted to the other side of the table. His hands were tied behind his back. He wasn't going anywhere.

His wife, her labia had these enormous piercings. They were pulled to a painful limit and fastened to the table on one side. Her nipples, also with enormous piercings, were stretched to their limit and fastened to the other end of the table. She also had her hands tied behind her back. She also, was not going anywhere.

As a crowd gathered at the party, drinks in one hand, hors d'oeuvres in the other, I began to fist them one at a time. Valentine narrated like a sportscaster giving play-by-play, and the crowd cheered as I went deeper and deeper into the two of them.

At times, I alternated between them. Other times, I did them both at the same time with one arm buried in each ass. With each different thing, the crowd cheered. If you listened closely, you could hear the man and wife both, thanking the crowd. Or maybe they were thanking me. I'm not sure.

I managed to get almost elbow deep in both of them, which still boggles my mind that something like that is anatomically possible. I know how the body is arranged and put together. It just doesn't seem possible without some kind of serious health problem after.

The wife was a trooper. She matched her husband inch-for-inch and didn't cry uncle until I started to get more vigorous with my thrusts. I eased off on her and soon gave her a rest. She earned her a nice ovation from the crowd as they released her.

The husband wasn't giving up so easy. I gave him some rather forceful action until I saw his cock - which never actually got erect or it might have ripped the restraint off - twitch and spew a big load of cum onto the table. I held my fist in him all the way like that while his orgasm subsided and the crowd cheered. When they released him, he had tears in his eyes.

As impossible as this seemed, both were quite happy about the experience. They loved it and were already volunteering to do it again, maybe with the crowd getting a turn. I could only shake my head.

The Happy Hand Part 2: Discussion

If I've said it once, I've said it a bunch of times. I think fisting is one of the most intimate things two people can do. Any two people can fuck. But the trust, communication and intimacy is on a whole different level when you allow someone to shove their whole hand inside your body.

One of the most interesting aspects is that everyone is different. Okay correction. Everyone IS different even without a fist in them. But with a fist in them, the subtle differences in each person's body are so pronounced that it is on a whole different level.

First, the trick to going in is so different with each person. Once you get four fingers in, you can feel the tissue stretch. You can feel every muscle, every curve, every bump, every ridge. You can feel their bone structure. You can feel how nervous they are. Or, how much they trust you. You can feel how turned on they are. Or not. You feel everything.

I get asked often which I prefer, vaginal or anal fisting, fisting men or women. That's really a tough choice. They all have their pleasures, for me, as the one doing the fisting. I like it all!! But, if I had to choose, I'd have to say vaginal fisting. I'm a giver. My favorite thing to do in bed is make women cum!! The inside of a pussy has soooooo many ways to make her cum. I think, possibly, as many as on the outside. Maybe more.

Each vagina is so different, just as each woman is different. First, the geography. Her outer labia. How full and plump is it? Is it hairy, or smoothly waxed (my favorite)? Then the inner labia. I love full lips. Aesthetically, they are mesmerizing to look at. They are art to me. When I go down on a woman, I can stay on her lips forever. Just licking every little fold of tissue. Sucking on them. Squeezing them between my lips and pulling them gently.

But functionally, they can present a challenge. Not enough lube and you'll be shoving them inside, which can't be pleasant. The hood. The more of a hood she has, the more sensitive her clit might be because the increased hood size keeps the clit from being touched as often. Think about how much contact a penis has in your pants all day. A clit hood protects the clit from the same kind of contact. The less contact it gets, the more you'll wake it up when you push that hood back. The more sensitive it is, the more fun you can have.

The opening is not really round. Well, most of them aren't. They look round, but they're more oblong shaped, top to bottom (with her on her back). It's kind of a hand-yoga challenge. The good stuff is on the top (g-spot for example) and the bottom (p-spot), not so much side-to-side. Yet, the easiest way to go in is with the hand sideways. I like to wiggle my finger across her g-spot as I use all four fingers. It probably doesn't do anything for her when I do that. No one has ever said, "Oh, I like that." She's probably thinking, 'Oh shit! He's about to fist me!' The finger thing probably doesn't even offer a distraction, but I try it anyway.

For some women, it is helpful to have an orgasm or two BEFORE I shove my big ol' hand into her. I personally think the biggest hurdle isn't that it won't fit; it's that she THINKS it won't fit and isn't relaxed. There are a few women that have a vaginal opening that is actually too small for success on the first attempt. That's actually the exception. They must relax and trust me though. Also, they must be relaxed enough with me to communicate well. I NEED information from her for this to work. If I'm not reading her body accurately, she has to be able to tell me. Having an orgasm (or two, or three) relaxes her in a manner that she's comfortable with and allows her to relax for us to continue.

When I have four fingers inside, I can get a feel for how I'll need to push the rest of my hand in. I use my middle finger to feel for the cervix. Later, I'll play with that. But going in the first time, I don't want to hit it. Banging the tip of the cervix, or cervical opening, usually isn't pleasant (at best) and can be painful for some women (at worst). Chances are good that if I hit it too hard, she'll clamp up and I won't be going in. It'll also be quite the turnoff, often times.

I also use my finger tips to feel how much room there is above her urethral sponge. The vagina can be quite deep - that doesn't seem to matter whether or not she's had children. The shape and size of the inside of a vagina also doesn't seem to depend on the size of the girl, either. The largest vaginal cavity I've ever met was in one of the smallest women I've ever met and the smallest was in (probably) the biggest woman I've ever been with.

When she's ready, I fold my thumb towards the palm and push, still careful not to bang her cervix. As I push in, I can feel her structure stretch - the muscles, her bones. I listen to her. She will give me the clues I need. "More." "Easy." Sometimes, there's an "Oh shit!!" Sometimes, a moan or a gasp. A sharp inhale of air. A dramatic increase in her breathing. As I push past the tightest point, I slightly turn my hand clockwise (using my right hand, with her on her back). By turning my hand 1/4, once in, my fingertips will be right there on her g-spot. If one finger, or two, stroking her g-spot is nice, imagine all four fingers, strongly pressed against it.

As soon as I push past the widest part of my hand, I STOP MOVING for a moment. I give her a chance to adjust. Especially the first time, having a fist inside is a little overwhelming and she'll need to wrap her brain around it. Many women have never experienced the "full" sensation. Some say it is life changing. And a PERSON inside them like this is very different from a toy or some kind of object, even a toy that mimics a fist.

For many, it is a sexual high like nothing else. The connection is so intimate that nothing compares forever after. I can literally feel her heartbeat around my wrist, and she can usually feel mine. Some women can orgasm right there, without moving any more than that, because of the intense physical stimulation combined with the emotional bond. THAT is something I love.

Once in, I gently "look around". Get the feel for the geography. There's a nice spot above the urethral sponge. You have the "dip" where the g-spot is. Then above that is a smooth (usually) patch of terrain that is very sensitive. It NEVER gets touched unless her man has a very long and freakishly strong and curved penis. Imagine the first time you stroke that!! I don't know if there's even a name for it. But rub it gently and watch her reaction. (grins).

Once she has gotten used to my hand inside her, I slowly start to move in and out. Some women like me to rotate my hand left and right. Some, do not. A large part of the sensation of fisting has to do with where the bones are in my hand and wrist. Rotating those bones stretches the vaginal opening in ways that toys and / or a penis never does. For some women, the actual vaginal opening has never been stimulated that way before and it is intense!! Some women who do not like rotating my wrist tell me it's that the bones apply an impact sort of pressure to her bones. Others say that the stretching of her vaginal opening like that is uncomfortable. Remember, the opening seems more vertically oblong in it's natural ability to give and stretch for this. So, horizontal pressure can go either way on the pleasure scale.

One of my absolute favorite things to do is slowly "roll" my knuckles across her g-spot. Just turning my wrist a little, slowly side to side - nothing else - bumps the knuckles over that sponge and... Well, I'm told that is unbelievable. It's also usually effective to roll my wrist forward and back, stroking the urethral sponge vertically (think of the same motion as slowly, gently knocking on a door only with the hand inverted). A variation is to apply pressure as I use either motion. Not every woman likes that. And some state that it's the wrong kind of pressure. But some, will squirt like fountains and lose their ability to speak coherently. That's why I try it. I love the look on a woman's face when she's having an "OH MY FUCKING GOOOOOOOOOODDDDD" moment. For me, that is almost as good as having one myself. Correction. Sometimes, it's better. What can I say? I'm a giver.

Another place that often gets overlooked is the P spot. On the bottom of her vagina (with her laying on her back), the tissue between her vagina and anus can be very sensitive. Like a lot of the inside, it doesn't get stimulated very often during intercourse and even when a lover uses their hand, this wall usually gets overlooked in favor of the g-spot. It's generally a more smooth surface. So usually, there are no landmarks to guide your exploration. Potentially, the whole surface can be sensitive. I use my fingertips to find the spots that are most sensitive and then I can close my hand to use my knuckles to stroke them harder, or with more pressure.

In women right there, there is the perineal sponge, at the perineum, between the vaginal canal and anal canal. The perineal sponge actually has erectile tissue and swells like a penis to help make a vagina tighter. It is sensitive like a penis and possibly contributes to vaginal orgasms via intercourse. You can stimulate it with your fingers on the back or bottom of the vagina and actually bring a woman to orgasm just as effective as stimulation to her g-spot. Many women go their entire lives and never have an orgasm from this, because, let's face it, the front side of things gets all the attention. Masturbating, it's hard to crank the wrist around to stroke it. Most men are aiming for the clit and g-spot, because you know, that's where we're told the magic happens. So, this area gets ignored a lot.

Ladies, DO. YOUR. KEGELS. One of the bits that gets the benefit is the perineal sponge. It's important to have a strong pelvic floor. It helps prevent incontinence when you get older or after you have kids. It'll help you ejaculate. BUT, the immediate and more noticeable and most happy reason is that Kegels will make sex feel infinitely better.

If you're coordinated, slide a well-lubricated finger (or two) inside her ass as you explore the P-spot. Find your fingers inside the vagina and rub them together through the tissue. I have been told that sensation is what makes a DP amazing. This spot is one of the reasons that many women orgasm from anal play. Combined with the rarity of it being stimulated, and the unique way it stimulates, it can offer many, many "OH MY GOD" moments.

Before I talk about playing with the cervix, I need to emphasize the importance of hand care. Before you slide your hand inside a person, an extreme manicure is a necessity. I don't mean trim the nails to where they're even and they look nice. I mean, there can be NO jagged edges. NO sharp edges. It has to be completely smooth. Not just the fingertips, but the sides of the fingertips and every surface of the hand. All calluses have to be removed. Guys, imagine a hangnail rubbed forcefully across the head of your penis. Yeah. It's like that. Some people wear gloves to help with this issue, and some will "pad" the inside of the gloves to aid in preventing a scratch. Well, that's fine. But if you have a hangnail, it will still be felt through the glove.

I personally prefer to not wear gloves. I want the intimacy. I want to FEEL the person I am fisting. Every heartbeat. Every detail of the inside of their body. I want to FEEL all that as well as the intimate connection of skin on skin. For me, it is orgasmic to feel another person so intimately. That emotional connection, to me, is greater than any orgasm for my own body. I have experienced about all the physical pleasures a man can have. Once discovering emotional and mental orgasmic bliss, I am now far more driven by that. That's just me though. On the receiving end, the reviews are mixed on whether a glove makes any difference. Some prefer it; some prefer not.

Okay, that said, let me move on. The cervix can be either very nice or very NOT nice to play with. Reviews are about half and half. Of those who didn't like it, some say it didn't feel very pleasurable. Some say it actually hurt. Some say it is just too weird. Of those who have not had children, the "too weird" was more common. Of the ones who have had children, some said it reminded them of pregnancy or childbirth in some way and it was not enjoyable. For both of those, the mental discomfort was a wall that prevented us from finding out if it physically felt good or not. Usually though, if a woman trusts me enough to shove a fist into her, she's probably not too freaked out about the idea of me touching her cervix and seeing what that's like.

There are quite a few women that have intense DEEP orgasms from cervix stimulation. Did I say "intense"? Did I say "DEEP"? Holy cow!! I mean, VERY intense and VERY deep orgasms. The full body kind. The kind that need aftercare before you can continue. The first time a woman feels that kind of orgasm, that also changes her life. It is life-changing in a way that is different from the way squirting is life changing. Or the first time they experience an anal orgasm. Those are all amazing. But what they experience from a cervical orgasm is apparently the most amazing of all.

Beverly Whipple and Barry Komisaruk, who is a psychologist at Rutgers, and one of my personal heroes, have investigated the vagus nerve and deep vaginal orgasms in women who have had spinal cord injuries. The spinal cord damage causes a lack of feeling in their lower extremities, thus not allowing them the ability to have orgasms by conventional means. The vagus nerve doesn't travel through the spinal cord, however. Deep, penetrative sexual activities that affect the cervix and stimulate the uterus trigger orgasm via this nerve. These women can have and feel the orgasms wonderfully.

At the other end, the vagus nerve begins in the throat and mouth. It travels through the chest, connects the heart and lungs, travels down through the digestive system, and ends up with a connection to the uterus and cervix. If deep, intense orgasms are possible in women with spinal cord injuries because of this major nerve system, then why not the same results when anything along the system is stimulated? Specifically, the mouth and throat. But also, women report experiencing these deep, full body orgasms from breathing exercises, singing and vigorous exercise. All of these are connected via the vagus nerve.

There's a guy right now all over the internet with a course in the 6 different kinds of orgasms a woman can have. ALL the women's empowerment coaches and sexuality life coaches and women's sexuality life coaches have all been pushing his course for $299-$599 a download. It has me screaming at my computer. His course talks about the 8 different kinds of orgasm that a woman can have, including tantric orgasms and mental orgasms. I keep thinking, "8? Just 8? There are 8 different kinds just inside the vagina!!" Ugh!! SMH

Moving on.

There are three things that I do with my hand inside her. First, I gently caress the cervical opening with my fingertips. Very gently to acclimate her to the sensation.

Once she is used to that, I push a finger into the opening and attempt to finger her cervix. The muscles there, pound for pound, are some of the strongest in the human body. They're designed to push a bowling ball through an opening the size of a soda bottle. Many times, the opening is too tight, even for a finger. Pressure to push inside is often too much and can be painful. With women who have not had children, this is more common. If I can get even the tip of my finger inside and can gently fuck her cervix with it, it can be quite pleasurable. Like I said, some women have DEEP, intense, full-body orgasms from this. If nothing else, it can be just pleasurable enough for a "Wow!" gasp.

The third thing I do is to use my fingertips to "suck" and pull on the cervix. Not hard, but firmly. The cervix doesn't always have enough to grip to do that, and it is difficult to grab on to even when there is enough for that. It doesn't always cause an orgasm. But, it can be very pleasurable, in a "that's weird" sort of way.

If nothing else, it will also create great circulation in the uterus and immediately cure her menstrual cramps for the month. Jus' sayin', if that applies to you.

Something that HAS given a few orgasms is when I insert a bullet vibrator inside my hand as I fist her. That, by itself, can be awesome. Once inside, I can touch that vibrator on things that have NEVER felt a vibrator before. All those places that rarely get stimulation, imagine the extra stimulation of a vibrator!! Particularly, I like using the tip of that bullet on the cervical opening. Sometimes, where I couldn't get a finger to open her up, the bullet does, and I slide that just barely inside the opening… Once they can form words again, I'm told that is quite nice. (grins)

Word of caution though, don't fully insert ANYTHING into the cervix. First, that opening can tighten up at any second and you'll need major surgery to remove whatever is in there. Second, there is a risk of infection from anything going in there. Just letting you know.

And, either before the hand is inside or after, don't forget to touch and stroke the sides of the inside of the vagina. They NEVER get touched like this. Lightly brushing my fingertips around them can be orgasmic. I'm told that the inside of the vagina is so sensitive in all those places that NEVER get touched that they can even feel the hair on the back of my hand as I move around. I talk a lot about having an exploration session. THIS is one of the coolest things to discover in that exercise.

BTW, I have had the pleasure of fisting a few women who have had a complete hysterectomy. Where the cervix WAS left a nub in one woman and a small pocket, or dip, in another in the back of their vaginal cavity. The one with the nub enjoyed me touching it and she said "thumping" it lightly with my fingers gave her a wonderful orgasm. The other one, wasn't impressed with anything I did to her dip. No pain or discomfort or anything like that. Just no thrills, either. The others were just as mixed between nubs and dips and pleasure or not.

Anal fisting a woman is very different from fisting a man. For those who enjoy it, it feels great for both of them. But for the women I've done this with, it seems to have an added sense of accomplishment that men are less excited about. With a man, I can say, "Wow! You just had my whole hand inside your ass!" And they're like, "And?" Women are like, "I KNOW, RIGHT? THAT WAS AMAZING!!" I like that. It's a greater challenge because women's bodies are smaller. So, women seem to be far more excited about the accomplishment when they get there.

Women (who have never been anally fisted) seem to be quite content with a slow, methodical process that ends with the desired results. Men, often are in a hurry. They tend to get impatient. Impatience can result in an injury. Impatience can result in giving up before any real progress is made. Women seem to be more determined to make progress and eventually achieve the goal, even if it takes a while. That's just an observation of mine based on my own experience and nothing else.

To go from never before to being able to ENJOY a fist in her ass, can take a while. It takes regular, frequent training to get there. Start with one finger, then two, etc. Slow and steady. Lots of lube. Lots of foreplay. Alternate with toys and fingers and cock. And don't forget your tongue. Easting her ass can open her up better than anything else. For some, it can be as orgasmic as eating her pussy.

Once a woman enjoys anal sex, you might be able to just jam your dick in there any ol' time you want. But to work up to a fist takes patience. Lots of patience. It won't happen the first time you try. Maybe not even the tenth or twentieth. It might take months. And once accomplished, it takes regular practice to keep it pleasurable or you may have to start over. The anus DOES return to it's normal size and tightness soon after even the most vigorous fisting - IF you didn't rush things, IF you are patient about building up to a fist, IF you are regular with practice as opposed to every once in a while. Do your Kegels. Seriously. The same exercise that keeps things tight, exercises the muscles and allows for greater flexibility. The greater the flexibility, the more they can stretch open, survive and return to normal.

My ex wife was the greatest partner for anal fisting. I still miss fisting her ass. When we started off, she had only had anal sex twice and didn't particularly enjoy it either time. I started slowly and gently. I used toys and fingers combined with lots of going down on her while I did so. She had her first anal orgasm with two fingers in her ass and my tongue working on her clit. She had her second one with my tongue in her ass.

After that, her world changed. She became obsessed with all things anal. She had no idea that we'd eventually be fisting her ass - probably didn't even cross her mind. But after that first anal orgasm, her driving thought was, "Let's try THAT in my ass." A trip to the grocery store had an entirely different meaning after that. I'm looking at the grocery list; she was looking at various bottles and objects, thinking, "I wonder if..." We filled plastic bottles and jars with marbles and a bullet vibrator. We filled them with water, alternating hot and cold. We tried all kinds of bottle shapes and sizes, all of them had her saying, "WOW, THAT WAS AMAZING!!"

It wasn't long and I scarcely touched her pussy any more. I went down on her to warm her up. But, she was waiting for the anal play. THAT was what got her off. That's what she wanted more than anything. When we worked up to a fist - a process that only took about two months practicing every other day - she was in heaven. THAT was it. THAT feeling was what she had wanted all her life. It was the most extreme sensation she could imagine. I'm sure it felt amazing. But just as amazing was the sense of accomplishment of the amazing thing she could do. There were times, just the suggestion of fisting her ass while I rubbed her butt gave her an orgasm.

Inside, there really isn't any trick to it. You go in the same way as vaginal fisting. One finger, two, three, then fold the thumb into your palm and push. Usually, you have to push a little harder. With the anus, there's definitely a sphincter that has to be forced open and then it kinda "pops" closed around the wrist. That sphincter is what makes it tight and what makes it a challenge.

And once inside, it is tight on the wrist. VERY tight. You can lose feeling in your hand. One thing that works well for that is to pull the hand back out slightly, which pulls on that sphincter. That will help relieve the circulation issue in the hand, but it also seems to be quite pleasurable for the person being fisted.

Some like deeper strokes in and out. But everyone that I've fisted anally liked the sensation of the sphincter being pulled out a little. Some like rotating my hand; others did not. Most were quite content with a gentle fucking in and out, gradually building the speed and intensity. For women, it helps to have a vibrator on her clit. But some have plenty of orgasms just with the anal stimulation. My wife loved it when I pushed as deep as I could go (sometimes half way up my forearm) and then pulled almost all the way out, then back deep again. Very slow and steady, in and out, faster and faster as she approached orgasm.

She was a very orgasmic woman from anal play and it was from anal fucking that she squirted the first time. Once we started with anal fisting, we had to consider the pool before we started because she would squirt buckets. At first, we used plastic garbage bags, usually, which also helped trap the EVOO we preferred to use as lube. Later, we started investing in puppy pads, which is, by far, the best things for squirting.

For men, it is also about the pleasure. The sense of accomplishment doesn't seem to be as much of a factor, though. It's almost like, "Sure. I can take that. What of it?" It still takes time and patience to work up to it. It still takes practice to maintain it. But because men are bigger, it seems to be a quicker process to achieve it. Men are definitely less cerebral and less emotional about it most of the time. Even if they like the connection and intimacy, that isn't what's going to get them off. They will truly have anal generated orgasms. I say it like that because orgasm is what takes place in the brain; not what happened with the body.

For women, orgasm makes much more sense to me because they are incorporating everything, every part of what's happening to their body, culminating in the cerebral event. It doesn't matter where or how on their body you are stimulating, the brain will orgasm when it feels good and it reaches the threshold. You get the brain involved, you can do pretty much anything to a woman's body and she can orgasm (generally speaking). That orgasm triggers a physical response of pleasure, such as squirting, or just a full body euphoria. THAT is what makes women such amazing creatures. It isn't just that you made their clit happy. Their entire BEING is happy and involved in the orgasm.

With men, during intercourse or oral sex, the cerebral event is generally just the opposite. It is usually triggered by the physical pleasure. Men generally are less cerebrally involved in the sex act. But when they are being fisted, I think this may be the same as women. It's still about the physical pleasure.

And, they are less impressed with being able to take a fist. But the men I have fisted have had orgasms that are more full bodied, euphoric, with less of a visible physical response. Many men, when being fisted, don't even get erect. They often don't ejaculate. Some don't even have any precum. In fact, quite a few that I have fisted told me that stimulating their cock would be a distraction from the pleasure of the fisting. Some like it, but they have to compartmentalize the two sensations to be able to enjoy either of them.

Men also seem to enjoy the ol' in 'n' out motion. Deep, then almost out, then deep. A couple have wanted my hand coming completely out, then back in forcefully. Fewer men that I've fisted enjoyed rotating my hand/wrist. Anatomically, there's no reason that men or women would be any different with that, except for maybe how it applies pressure to the prostate. Just a theory. The men tend to prefer it more "enthusiastic" and "vigorous" than women. Again, just my experience.

One last thing I want to say is about D/s relationships. Fisting is often seen as a dominant act. It is easy to think that the FISTEE is the sub and the FISTER is the Dom. I don't think that's necessarily true. Sure, sometimes it definitely will be like that. But, it doesn't have to be. I'm a giver. My entire motivation in sex is to GIVE pleasure. Sometimes, I do that from a dominant role. Other times, I can quite submissive. It really depends on the energy between myself and the other person.

As a dominant, I'm fisting the person. As a submissive, I'm fisting the person. The act doesn't change. Giving pleasure doesn't change. The D/s roles only change because of the energy - not the act of fisting them. So, if you're a Dom and you want to try being fisted, I don't think it changes your role. If you're a sub and you want to do some fisting, I don't think it changes your role. D/s is about energy and the relationship, not the particular activity. Just my opinion.

The Happy Hand Part 3: More Stories

Story 3

My wife came into the living room and put her arms around me from behind the couch. She'd been in the bathroom for an eternity getting cleaned out and then taking a nice, warm bath. She smelled intoxicating. She was ready. "Tonight's the night," she said softly in my ear.

I turned my head and looked her in the eyes. "You think so?"

"Let's just say, I feel optimistic." We had been trying for a couple of months to get my fist in her ass. We'd managed some large toys and I almost got there a couple times, but it hadn't quite happened yet.

I met her in the bedroom. She was already naked and had assumed the position on the bed. We always started with a sensual massage of her petite body. A warm, loving touch head to toe to relax her. When she was ready for more, she'd flip over onto her back for me to go down on her. One thing that was so perfect about her was her non-verbal communication. I'd get an "Oh, yeah" and "Yes" when I first touched her pussy with my mouth. But after that, she couldn't form words. Like a language all it's own, her sounds of pleasure told me everything I needed to know. I knew when I was giving her what she wanted or needed and I knew when she was cumming. Really, she made my job so much easier. I loved that.

After an orgasm, out came the toys. I used a vibrator on her clit with one hand and the fingers of my other hand inside her. Basically, I was priming the pump, so to speak. Once she squirted the first time, she was like a faucet that couldn't be turned off. Once she started squirting, she was ready for the anal play. A good squirt and even before she caught her breath, she turned over and assumed the position, ass up, face down.

I listened to her breathing smooth out as I rimmed her. She moaned in approval. Sometimes, that was enough to bring her to orgasm again. This time it was. With her orgasm, I escalated. Next came fingers. One. Two. Three. Four. By the time I had four fingers inside her, she often came again. This time, even before she could reload, I folded my thumb into my palm and began to push. I applied the Hitachi to her clit. I tried to time the final push with her orgasm. As she moaned distinctly, I pushed hard and could feel her sphincter slide over my hand to the wrist. She screamed and her whole body trembled uncontrollably.

"You okay?"

She fought to form the words between hard breaths. "Green," she whispered. "Green. Oh my God, green" After a few moments of me not moving a muscle, she managed to follow with, "That is the most incredible thing I have ever felt."

After a few minutes allowing her body to adjust, I slowly began to fuck her ass with my hand. As soon as I began to move, she came again. I paused this time as it subsided. She nodded her head and I began to move again. Within seconds, she came again. This time, she squirted a flood between her legs and her body tensed so tight that I became painfully aware that I was losing feeling in my hand. As the orgasm subsided, I began pulling my hand out.

"NOOOO!!!" she screamed and I stopped. Right there, with my thumb still inside her. my wrist managed to get some quick relief. She reached around and grabbed my arm Forcefully, with a grunt, she shoved my hand back inside her and began thrusting back against me. I fucked her ass harder and she squirted over and over and over, with loud moans and indecipherable words screamed into the bed. After about fifteen minutes, she screamed one last time and I could tell she was done. She rocked forward on her knees, slowly pulling my hand out of her in one motion. She rolled over on her back and was silent as she fought to catch her breath.

"I'll be so sore tomorrow," she whispered, "but I already want to do that again." She grabbed me and pulled me down on her. She kissed me so passionately that I knew I'd taken her to a wonderful new place. I could feel the sweat on her body against me. I could feel her heart beating hard in her chest. Her arms held me tight against her as she slowly began to come down. After an eternity (it seemed), she whispered "Thank you."

From that night, I fisted her ass at least once a week for the remainder of our relationship. Even after we began to fail as a couple, she negotiated blowjobs for fisting her ass. Every other act of love or affection was gone, but she NEEDED that. Even though we were falling apart, that was our last string holding us together. Sigh.

Story 4

Bama and I on FetLife. Quickly, we REALLY hit it off well. Quickly, we moved up to phone calls. Quickly, we planned a road trip for her to come visit me. All the while, she insisted there was no way that my fist would fit inside her. She actually laughed at the idea. I think she really just wanted to get laid. I don't think she really expected much beyond that. After all, a lot of guys talk a big game. How many really know anything? She also went on and on about what a sub she was and that she knew she would spend a large chunk of the weekend trying to take all of my cock down her throat.

She arrived and before she could even say hello, I pushed her to her knees. I was wearing gym shorts, commando, and I pulled them down to release my cock. She knew what to do and began sucking my cock in and out. She tried to put her hands on it, but I told her "No. Just your mouth." The second time, I told her to undo her pants and masturbate as I fucked her mouth. But, I forbade her from cumming. Slowly, I fucked her mouth for a while, shoving my cock all the way down. To her credit, she is the only woman who has taken my entire dick down her throat on the first attempt.

After a few minutes, she turned her head and my cock slid out of her mouth. "May I cum?" she asked.

"Soon," I answered and put my cock back in her mouth. I fucked her mouth harder, burying the entire length down her throat. I held it there with a firm grip on her head and gave her permission.

When I thought her orgasm had faded, I let her up for air. I put my dick back in my shorts and pulled her to her feet. "Hi," she whispered and smiled.

"Hi," I replied softly and smiled too. "Come on in."

She grabbed her bag and brought it to the bedroom, setting ti down by the closet door. "Where's your bathroom? I've needed to pee since about Chattanooga." We laughed and I pointed to the bathroom. While she relieved herself, I lit a couple candles and got some puppy pads. I laid a couple out on the floor at the foot of the bed and a couple more on the end of the bed.

When she returned, I motioned her to the end of the bed. I kissed her lightly as I started taking her clothes off, all the while looking her in the eyes. She didn't know what to say yet. She'd been in the apartment less than 15 minutes and had been throatfucked, had an orgasm and was now naked in my bedroom.

Naked, I spun her around and bent her over the bed. I reached under her and found her soaked pussy. I began rubbing her clit firmly as I lightly ran my hand over the cheeks of her ass. I swatted her hard on the right cheek as I removed my hand from her pussy. I applied the hand again for a few minutes, but removed it before swatting her left cheek. Each time, she moaned, "Yeah!" followed by a soft, "Thank you." I swatted each cheek again this way and then began to finger her from behind.

One finger, two fingers, three fingers. I fucked her that way while I still rubbed her clit underneath with my other hand. Soon, I began the "come hither" motion inside her with two fingers and she thanked me with a very nice squirt that hit the end of the bed and splattered all over my legs. I continued until she squirted again. Once she did that, I could feel that she was relaxed enough for more. I slipped a third finger back inside her and kept fucking her slowly. Soon, a fourth finger. She came again with four fingers inside her and my other hand still rubbing her clit, releasing a new flood of squirt and an "Oh FUCK!"

I used four fingers for a few minutes and she came again, squirted again and her knees trembled. "Hold on, dear." I told her. I reached for the KY with the hand that had been on her clit and applied it the right hand, as it continued to slowly fuck her. She felt the coolness of the lube on my hand and I think she knew what was coming next, but was unable to stop it. I folded my thumb into my palm and pushed my hand inside her.

I thought she was going to lose it. Her legs shook. Her breathing elevated instantly. And she squirted so much that it challenged the puppy pads. She moaned so loud I am sure my neighbors heard her and then squirted again. Gently, I began rotating my hand back and forth, rolling my knuckles across her g-spot. She moaned loudly again and squirted again. "Aaaaahhhhh FUUUUUCCCKK!!" I began to fuck her faster and harder. I shoved my full fist in and pulled it almost out, back in and back out. Over and over. I lost count of how many times she squirted. I just knew my legs were soaked and my feet were in a puddle.

One more strong orgasm and I held my fist deep inside her, not moving, as she cooled down. When I slowly slid my hand out, she collapsed on the bed and began catching her breath. "Okay. I stand corrected. It fit nicely."

"Told ya it would."

We laughed. "You earned a sammich, but you'll have to wait for me to take a nap." She climbed all the way up on the bed and began fumbling for the comforter. "I'll also finish that blowjob and clean up the mess. OH MY GOD!! I have never squirted that much!!"

I snickered. I admit, I'm cocky. But this went much better than expected. She made good on finishing the blowjob later and then we went to dinner.

Story 5

Another time Bama came to visit, we attended a squirting demonstration. Geared towards beginners, so it was a little boring for us. But what made it more interesting was to see a woman squirting right before my eyes. Like, live porn.

After, the leader of the demonstration asked if anyone else wanted to share in the show. Bama and I raised our hands. The leader invited us up front and we went.

Bama responds best bent over. So, I bent her over the table. The table was soaked from the previous demonstration and I pushed her down right in it. Later, she told me that was so gross and disgusting, but it turned her on like nothing ever had. (grins)

I lifted her skirt and swatted both cheeks of her plump ass a couple times, which also seems to jump start her flow of juices. There was a collective "Oh!" from the audience when the "SMACK" came. I knelt down behind her and grabbed her panties right along her ass crack and RIPPED them open so her ass was fully exposed. I heard her moan softly. The audience let out a huge collective gasp. A few people actually applauded. LOL

I slipped two fingers in and began stroking her g-spot. In moments, she was soaking the floor, and possibly the feet of the people in the front row. The audience gasped again. Then, without any warning, I shoved my fist inside her and began fucking her hard. I don't know how many times she squirted. I only know that she stole the show.

After, she was the most popular girl in the room as people came up to her like a rock star. They asked about the squirting. But mostly, they asked about the fisting. Her answer, "I recommend it."

Story 6

I will never forget Billie Marie. Such a tiny little woman. Such an absolutely cavernous vagina though. I swear I could have parked a car in there. I'm not sure she was even 5' tall and was tiny in build. Not bony thin; just slender and fit. Perfectly proportioned; just tiny. Yet, by far the largest vagina I have ever met.

I was still kinda new to fisting or I probably would have turned her into a research project. Something like, "Let's see if THIS will fit in there, honey." I fisted her pussy almost to my elbow and I think she could have easily taken more. I was the one who backed off, though. I still think she could have taken both of my fists - EASILY!! In that moment, I was so excited that I didn't think of it. Hindsight. Sigh.

I'm not even sure she knew that her pussy was "special". I really don't think she did. But it was. Oh, it was. I still fantasize about her. In my fantasy, I have my fist inside her. AND my cock, and I am jerking my cock inside her. Something like that. I saw that in a video once and immediately thought of her. It was just that one night. But, she is one of two women that I still think about many years later. I will never forget her.

Story 7

Then there was SOB (aforementioned in some of my other stories). She's the one who made these wild cat noises when she was aroused and came.

A friend was visiting, sleeping on the couch one time. The next morning, I'm in the kitchen making coffee. He was sitting at the breakfast bar very quiet. I asked him what was up.

"Man," he started. "I want to know what the hell you do to a woman that makes her make CAT noises like that."

I laughed. I'm sure, without an explanation, it can be rather disturbing. I know it took me a few times before I could continue with the sex without cracking up. Before I could explain, my friend went on.

"'Cause see, I want to know to make sure I NEVER do that to a woman."

She is the only woman who has had both my fists in her pussy. That was a visual I have mixed feelings about. It was a borderline freakshow, yet, a freakshow I couldn't stop watching. One that I couldn't stop performing. I mean, in videos that looks amazing. In front of me, it was wild. I fuck that pussy. I eat that pussy. I don't want it ruined, ya know.

And just the visual is a little disturbing in real life. I don't know why it was like that with her and not with Billie Marie or anyone else. Maybe because we had a long term relationship. We did one in her pussy and one in her ass a couple times, but somehow that just didn't seem as freaky. Another time, we ALMOST got both my fists in her pussy while a girlfriend fisted her ass. But, that found her limit and I was only able to do one. Next time, dear. Next time.

SOB was a squirting phenom. I don't even know how it was possible to squirt the sheer volume and force she squirted with. But each time she squirted, it was so overwhelming of an orgasm that she needed a few moments to reload. With my fist inside her, she didn't get that moment. As huge as her pussy was, it still required a little work to extract my hand from her after an orgasm. Many times, just that movement would cause another huge orgasm. So, I would usually just freeze while she collected herself. Sometimes though, just being passive-aggressive, I would fist her hard and fast when she was expecting me to freeze. She would be entirely in some other dimension. It was the only time she came and didn't make those crazy cat noises.

Story 8

As for men, I hadn't fisted a man since Valentine's fisting school. Then out of the blue, I was contacted by OTR, also from FetLife. He was in the neighborhood and asked if I had ever fisted a man. I admitted it had been a while, but I was open to it. I picked him up and brought him home to perform the deed. We warmed up with some massive toys and then I fisted him. Then I took him home. Kinda anti-climactic.

The thing is, OTR talks non stop. I mean, NON STOP. He doesn't get a lot of people interaction truck driving, ya know. So when he gets a human in his presence, he unloads every single thing he has been keeping to himself for the past month or so. I mean, NON STOP. Even as he has my fist, half way to the elbow rocking his colon, he is talking about his truck or his kids or the Dallas Cowboys or his dog or politics or a TV show he saw, or the other people he plays with and whatnot. It was mind blowing. Not how much of my fist he could take, but that he never shut up. Occasionally, he would grunt, "Oh yeah. Right there." But usually, he was going on 90 mph about nothing.

That is possibly one of the strangest things I've ever been a part of. Not the fisting, but that he just kept talking so much and so fast. I dare say, it MIGHT be weirder than clown sex or cat noises or that woman in Roane County fucking ALL her step-kids while their daddy watched and beat off in the closet. Might be.

Afterwards, I asked him if he enjoyed it. He gushed, "Oh, it was amazing!!"

"How would I know?" I asked.

"You couldn't tell?" he answered.

I didn't know what to say. So, I said nothing. He might not even be aware that he talks like that. NO. I couldn't tell. I'm not sure if I should have been able to tell or not. I mean, I feel like I SHOULD HAVE been able to. But then, he TALKED THE WHOLE TIME ABOUT EVERYTHING EXCEPT THE FIST IN HIS ASS! How was I supposed to notice? I mean, almost to my elbow, ya know? And he's going on and on about this truck he got a great deal on and how his son wrecked it. I was busy paying attention to the story. How on earth was I to focus on what I was doing, or how well he was enjoying it?

Anyway... OTR has been here a couple of times, and he will be back again at some point I'm sure. Football season is here. We need to do the whole, "How 'bout them Cowboys!" conversation.

Story 9

Contrary to how I probably sound on here, I am actually quite careful in my private life. I'm very careful about where my dick goes. I don't fuck on the first date. I might not even fuck on the third or fourth date. I wait until I know the relationship has possibilities.

Part of that actually doesn't have anything to do with the risk of STDs, although that IS a risk I try to keep to a minimum. No, as I'e gotten older, maybe starting in my early 40s, the emotional side of sex has come front-and-center. In my youth, I fucked around with wild abandon and damn the feelings. I can't do that anymore. I NEED the feelings. I MUST have the emotional and mental and spiritual connection or the physical connection CAN'T happen.

A woman won't even get wet if she's not feeling what she needs. My dick has become like that. At first, I thought it was E.D. You Know? Getting older, a smoker, too much sitting and not enough exercise. Made sense. But as my relationship with my wife was falling apart, I realized that wasn't it because with someone I connected with, my dick seemed to work just fine.

So, when you read these stories about my crazy life, remember, I'm not really a slut. I just play one on the internet. I used to be one. Before the internet and cell phones with cameras (thankfully). Not anymore though.

Back in the day though…

Right after I got my legendary apartment in Knoxville, I was still kind of a slut, but not as much. I broke up with SOB a few days later. Let's just say there was an unfavorable turn in the story and leave it at that. Okay?

So there I was, new to the place and I was having a slight pity party. And then, out of the blue, a neighbor knocked on the door.

She had seen me walking my dog and wanted to know if we could arrange a play date. I'd only been in the apartment a few days, but I thought I had seen her too. I said sure and invited her inside. Regina was a cute, little woman, about 35ish, with short red hair and lots of freckles. She seemed very shy. She spoke quietly and softly. Always had a smile. Always very, very polite.

A few days later, we met for our arranged play date. My dog in those days was Spud, a black and white beagle mix, probably named after Spuds MacKensie. I got him from a friend who was being sent overseas for a reason I can't discuss, and because the dog was so old, he wasn't able to take him. Sadly, the poor old dog passed a couple of months after this.

Anyway, we met at the dog park and just turned the dogs loose. Spud tried to play but he was so old that he didn't really do much. He still loved the grass and the sunshine though. Her dog, Angel I think she said, napped in the grass next to him.

Regina and I sat in the grass nearby and got to know each other. She seemed so reserved and… Well, polite. She was very nice and I liked her. She had a nice sense of humor and was very smart. And sitting there, wearing cut offs and a halter, I could see a body that I would love to see more of.

We went to dinner. We went to a movie. We went to see the Smokies play. I cooked dinner for her a couple of times. There was no hurry to get naked. I had a lovely time with her and always got some passionate, but nice, kissing when we parted for the evening.

One night, I was cooking dinner and we started talking about "the sex date". This was probably our 6th or 7th date by this point over about a 3 week span since she had first knocked on my door. Many people talk about the 3rd date being the sex date and we laughed that we had eclipsed that.

"Have you run out of patience with me?" I asked, half joking. I mean, With her being so polite and all, I expected her to be VERY conservative and she might appreciate the slow pace. I was ready. But, I was going slow out of respect for HER.

"Well frankly," she answered. "If you don't fuck me tonight, I'm going to move on. Preferably in the ass."

That caught me off guard. It took me a few minutes to get my voice back. "I was being patient because you seemed so nice," I answered.

"Ha!" she laughed. "A woman can't be polite in conversation and have slutty desires?"

I smiled. "Are you telling me you have some slutty desires?"

"Like you'd never believe," she replied. Her usual polite smile turned somewhat dark and dirty, and I loved it.

I almost burned dinner when she said that. I left everything on the stove to get cold and dragged her to the bedroom immediately. I almost ripped her clothes off in my haste to reveal her cute little body. The drapes matched the curtains, if you know what I mean, and I smiled big as I threw her down on the bed.

I went down on her and saw a perfectly trimmed, petite little pussy. As I licked it top to bottom, she threw her slender legs up over her shoulders to give me better access. That was the night I realized how obsessively I like a flexible woman who can do that.

I stopped for a second to drink in the visual, and looking me right in the eyes with all seriousness, she quietly stated, "I love it in my ass more than ALMOST anything else."

Well, I almost came right then. For this nice little reserved woman to say that, so slutty, it was incredibly hot. Seriously, maybe it was just her and the way she softly said it, but it was one of the hottest things a woman has every said.

"I'll get there soon," I promised and buried my face in her pussy. I tongued her clit and labia like I was trying to win a prize and soon, she came with a very UNreserved scream.

From there, I slipped a finger inside and began to stroke her g-spot. Then two fingers. Then three fingers. Even though, visually, her pussy LOOKED tiny, it seemed limitless as I slipped fingers inside her.

"Fist me," she moaned.

I was briefly frozen. I mean, that's just not the words you expect to hear from such a "nice" little woman. I looked up at her, surprised. She looked back at me and forcefully said, "Do it!"

I pushed my whole hand in with surprising ease and she moaned, "Yes!" It was a very tight fit. I couldn't believe it really went in so easily. But, she was loving it. She came and then came again and was bucking her hips for more.

I used my signature move of rolling my knuckles across her g-spot. She screamed and came so hard that it cut the circulation off in my hand. I had to pull my hand back or I really thought I'd lose it.

"No!" she hollered as I almost pulled out. Really, like a demon. I wasn't sure if her head was going to spin around or what. A little scared, I pushed my fist back in and began fucking her with it a little harder. Each time I pulled back, I rolled my knuckles across her g-spot again. And each time, she screamed uncontrollably.

After a few more orgasms, I realized that each time I pushed in, I was getting deeper and deeper. By now, I was halfway to my elbow and she was still begging for more. I was hitting bottom, so it seemed, but she was loving it.

Finally, I pushed in as deep as I could - two thirds of my forearm - and she came one last time. Her whole body tensed up and I think she stopped breathing for a full minute.

As her breathing returned to normal, I slowly slid my arm out of her. It was numb. It was soaked unbelievably just from her natural juices. I found a towel and stood over her, watching her get her wits back.

After all that, I had a hard on that would drive nails and was anxious to get into her little ass, as promised. She was like jelly though. I pushed her legs up and she managed to get them over her shoulders, but barely. I swear, I think she slept through most of it. Even back then, I wouldn't normally fuck a sleeping woman. But at that point, I'm not sure it mattered to me.

As I got close to cumming, she perked up and seemed to rally. A second wind, of sorts, and she had another orgasm. When I heard her scream, I couldn't hold back anymore and unloaded in her tiny little ass.

She was asleep before I even slipped out of her. I toweled off and laid down next to her. At first, I was admiring her body. Even asleep, she was smiling politely. After a few minutes, I pulled the covers up over us. Spud came in and went to sleep in his bed. I soon fell asleep too.

A couple hours later, Spud woke me up. In our lust, we had forgotten to take the dogs out. I fumbled through Regina's pants and found the key to her apartment. I went and got Angel, let the two of them pee and brought them back inside. I gave each of them a treat and they went into the bedroom, presumably to share Spud's bed.

I cleaned up the kitchen. Dinner was ruined, but I didn't care. I had the biggest smile on my face as I washed the dishes.

After, I went back into the bedroom. Even in the dark, I could see her freckled face, smiling. I eased into bed next her and pulled her to me. She moaned a little, but I don't think she actually woke up. Soon, I was asleep again.

What woke me the next morning was the feeling of someone moving my arm around. At first, I was too sleepy to investigate as weird as it was. But when I felt her curling my fingers into a fist and positioning herself for insertion, I woke with a start.

"Aren't you sore?" I asked.

She shook her head. "I masturbate with more intensity that what we did."

I just looked at her, trying to wrap my head around that. I propped myself up between her legs and shoved my hand into her. I couldn't believe she wasn't sore. But, she moaned as I entered her.

"More intensity?" I asked.

She nodded and threw her legs up over her shoulders, looking deep into my eyes. "Is this slutty enough for you? Still think I'm nice and reserved?"

I smiled. Slowly, I began to stroke her. Each time I pushed deep, she very quietly gasped and moaned, "Yes."

"I can't believe you can take it so deep," I said.

"I fuckin' masturbate with toys bigger than that," she cried. "MORE!!"

That stopped me momentarily. I mean, this woman was tiny. She had a tiny little pussy. Later, I had her prove her claim and I got to watch her masturbate with some of the biggest toys I'd ever seen. Scary, some of them, and the intensity she rode them was beyond belief. But on this morning, I built tempo, depth and gave it as much intensity as my arm could handle.

I was pounding her as hard as I could, and I was past half way to my elbow on some strokes before she cried mercy. I eased back and rolled my knuckles across her g-spot a few times. If there was ever a time when I thought her head would really spin around, that was it.

She grabbed my arm and held it in place as her hips pushed herself onto me one last time. This time her scream was almost a silent one as she came one last time. Again, I don't think she took a breath for a full minute. Slowly, I pulled out of her, leaving a gape that was startling for such a petite woman.

She groaned and rolled over. Within minutes, she was back asleep. I usually feel rather proud when I satisfy a woman so fully that SHE falls asleep after. But in this case, I was starting to get a weird vibe about this.

I took the dogs out. I made some breakfast. I checked my emails. Soon, I heard the shower running. I checked the bedroom and saw a bed that should make any man proud. Sheets everywhere, covered in our fluids. Yep. I was proud.

I got her clothes and took them into the bathroom. She had left the door open, so I went in unannounced. I laid the clothes on the counter next to the sink and got her my biggest, fluffiest towel. She didn't even know I was in there. I went back into the kitchen and refilled my coffee cup. I got her a cup, put it on the table next to the sugar and cream.

She hollered, "Thank you," from the bathroom when she saw her clothes and the towel. A moment later, she joined me at the table for coffee. There was that smile. And the shy, reserved woman was back.

"I can't believe you're not insanely sore," I told her.

She shook her head, still smiling. "I told you. I masturbate with toys that are much more intense."

"How much do you masturbate like that? How often?" I asked.

She snickered. "Enough that it will change your opinion of how nice I am."

"Got some slutty desires, do you?"

"Always," she said quietly.

It was Saturday. We spent most of the day together. That evening, she showed me her toy collection and then showed me what she does with them. She was right. Some of her toys made my arm look small. And the way she rode them was fucking scary. "Intense" was definitely the right word.

And hot.

Watching her fuck herself so hard with those HUGE toys was so fucking hot. After she came a few times, she bent over the bed and offered her ass to me again. I took it. She came another 2 or 3 times as I fucked her. And after I came, she laid back on the bed and fucked her pussy with an enormous dildo until she came a few more times. I could only watch.

This time, instead of going to sleep, she seemed to still have plenty of energy. We went to IHOP and had some dinner. I was still in awe that she wasn't too sore to walk. You had to see what I saw. It just didn't seem possible that she could survive such a thrashing so nonchalant. Every time I said something, she just laughed.

Well. Every good thing must come to an end. That weird vibe came back. Just a feeling that there was a secret a big as her toys and the secret was about to come calling in a huge way. Just a feeling. You ever get that about someone?

From what she said, she was masturbating like that at least twice a day, with one of the times replaced by my fist pounding her mercilessly on the nights we got together.

I knew Regina was a nurse. She showed up one morning in her scrubs on her way to work. She had that polite smile. She kissed me as she came in, but went right over to the dining room table. She pulled her bottoms down and bent over. "Care to fuck my ass so I can go to work full of cum?"

She didn't have to ask twice.

After, I asked if we were going to see each other that night. I mean, for the few weeks, we had established a bit of a routine.

She politely said, "No. Sorry. This is goodbye for now."

I'm sure I looked disappointed. She tilted her head. "Awwww... How long did you expect this to go on?"

I shrugged.

"I'm married. My husband travels and he'll be back this afternoon. He leaves again in a few weeks, though. Get together then?" She kissed me - politely - and left me standing there stunned.

There was never any hint of a husband. No wedding ring or band. Not even a mark from a wedding ring or band. When I went into her apartment to get Angel that night, I didn't notice anything suggesting there was a husband. But then again, I was half asleep. I had that weird vibe, but that was all, and as you know, "vibes" aren't always clear. All that we had talked about and all the time we had spent together. Not one word or even a hint.

I saw her walking her dog here and there. And I saw the husband walking the dog a few times. I never knew what to say to her. So, I simply waved awkwardly when I saw her. Her husband was a big guy with big hands and arms. I noticed that. And she was always smiling. I noticed that too. It was like a dirty little secret.

They moved before the next time the husband went out of town. Part of me was very disappointed. Part of me wasn't.